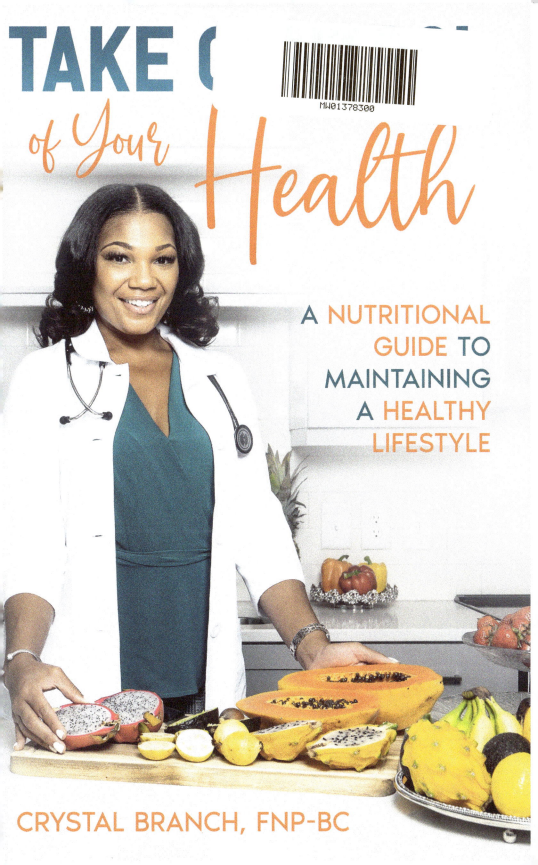

Table Of Contents

Acknowledgment

Introduction

Breakfast options 7

What is Gluten? 7

What is Agave? 8

What are the benefits of Agave? 12

What is GMO 11

Lunch: 12

Dinner: 14

Hypertension 27

Hypertension "High Blood Pressure" Diet Changes 34

Your Health & Water Intake 32

Carbonated Water 33

Cholesterol 37

Conclusion 42

Weekly Food and Exercise Log 43

List of Preservatives in Foods 91

References 93

Copyright

Printed in the USA by A2Z Books, LLC. Copyright by Crystal Branch. All rights reserved. This book or any portion thereof may not be reproduced or used in any manner whatsoever without the express written permission of the publisher or author except for the use of brief quotations in book review Printed in the United States.

First Printing
ISBN 978-1-955148-17-7
www.A2ZBookspublishing.net

Acknowledgment

I would like to Acknowledge My Savior Jesus Christ, who is the Head of My life. I want to thank my First Minister, My Husband Allen Howard for his amazing support. I would like to thank, My Publisher, my Photographer, My Editor that brought my vision to life I could not have done it without a team!
In life we don't know why things happen to us, but we have to remember that things happen for us! In order for you to walk into your gift, passion, calling, and Power God made within you, sometimes you have to be Pushed out of your comfort zone.
Be Encouraged and Keep Faith.

Love,
Crystal

Introduction

Have you ever wondered why you're killing yourself in the gym, working out but not seeing the results you desire?

Well, I'm here to inform you guys that the real work comes with the food that we eat.

This meal guide is intended to educate you on the basic foods you eat that could be causing your health and wellness goals to be stagnated.

You will discover simple adjustments and alternatives to implement in your diet to aid in your goals.

This 30-day meal guide will help you in your fitness journey but bear in mind this is not an overnight quick fix or fad. This is a lifestyle you must adopt to maintain a healthier version of yourself and make healthier choices.

With a lifestyle change, the term LIMIT is used to teach you how to use moderation instead of completely cutting things out of your diet cold turkey.

Lifestyle Change

- ✓ Limit fast foods
- ✓ Limit alcohol
- ✓ Limit sodas
- ✓ Limit juices
- ✓ Limit pork
- ✓ Limit beef
- ✓ Limit fried foods
- ✓ Limit starches

Lifestyle Change

- ✓ A diet with 2-4 servings of fruits a day.
- ✓ A diet full of 2-4 vegetables a day.
- ✓ A diet with a gallon of water a day.
- ✓ A diet with baked, broiled lean meats such as turkey, chicken, and fish.

Lifestyle changes with cooking oils:

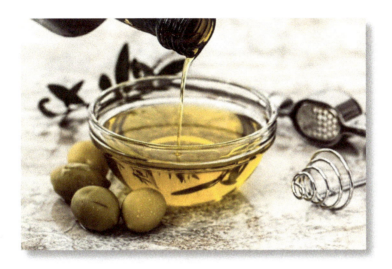

Make use of alternative healthy cooking oil; instead of using margarine, butter, and Crisco that increase cholesterol levels and put you at risk of heart disease such as heart attacks and strokes.

Use alternatives that are alkaline (low in acid). Any food that is low in acid decreases inflammation in the body. What is inflammation? It simply means soreness of muscles and aches as well as swelling within your body.

Cooking oil alternatives:

- Avocado oil
- Brazil nut oil
- Coconut oil (Not made for frying)
- Grapeseed oil
- Hemp seed oil
- Olive oil (Not made for frying)
- Sesame oil
- Walnut oil

Some Milk Alternatives:

Dairy has proven to cause inflammation in the body and is usually not easily digested in the human digestive system. Here are healthier choices of milk to consume:

- Coconut Milk
- Hemp Milk
- Walnut Milk
- Almond Milk

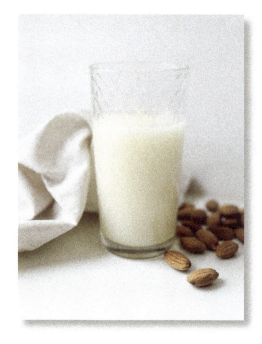

Snacks:

- Popcorn (sparingly)
- Plantain chips
- Any of these nuts and seeds:
    - Hemp seeds
    - Pistachios
    - Almonds
    - Cashews
    - Pecans
    - Sunflower Seeds

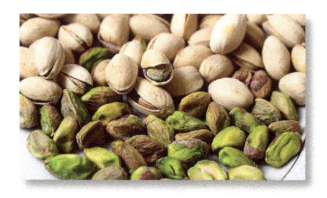

Seasonings contain a lot of preservatives such as hidden sodium and hidden sugars. Consider using healthier alternatives.

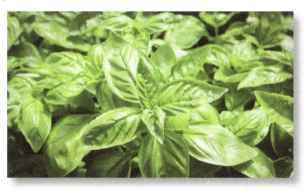

All-natural seasonings:

- Basil
- Bay Leaves
- Cloves
- Dill
- Oregano
- Parsley
- Thyme
- Pink Himalayan salt (use sparingly – one pinch)

Let's Get Started

Most of our calories come from the beverages we drink.

To accelerate your goal, it is good to drink at least 64 oz of water each day. To make things simple, drink a gallon of water a day.

When you drink water, it has no calories unlike when you drink beverages like orange juice, apple juice, and sodas.

Did you know that the average soda has about 150 calories and 44 grams of Sugar?

Fast Foods

Fast foods are prepared in such a way that we will never know all the ingredients it contains. We will also never truly know all the ingredients of the condiments we consume. Fast foods are packed with fillers to make our stomachs full without any nutritional value.

Most condiments are packed with preservatives and sugar for longer shelf life. Ever wondered why you feel sleepy after consuming fast foods? The reason is simply the lack of nutrients inside the food. When you are sluggish after eating it's due to preservatives that fail to fuel your body with the nutrients it needs. One of the many ways to attain your desired weight goal is to eliminate all fast food.

I understand that circumstances may arise that may require you to buy fast food or snacks such as when you are traveling or staying away from home. When you have to rely on fast foods due to circumstances, try to make better choices.

- Instead of pizza and a soda, choose a salad.
- Instead of fried nuggets, go for the grilled ones.
- Instead of eating fried chicken, mash potatoes, and a soda; choose grilled turkey or tuna wrap.
- Instead of eating cookies and chips for dessert; go for a piece of fruit, yogurt, or parfait.
- Instead of hamburgers, French fries, and soda; consider taking a salad.

There are numerous ways to make wiser choices. It's just up to you to make those healthy selections. So, you may ask yourself, what should I eat?

Here is a guide to accelerate your health and wellness goals!

Breakfast options

1. Gluten Free Oats with non-dairy milk

What is a gluten-free oat? They are simply oats that do not have gluten and Kamut is an excellent example of a gluten-free oat.

What is Gluten?

To understand what gluten-free oats mean, let's understand what gluten means. Gluten is found in most wheat grains and they are not easily digested by humans. Gluten is an elastic substance that sticks to the walls of your intestines when ingested and it causes inflammation (swelling in your intestinal wall).

For instance, instead of eating oatmeal for breakfast, eat Kamut oats.

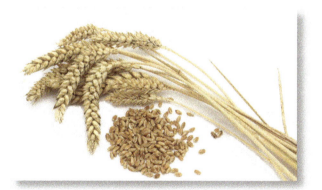

Items to eat in the morning:

Use 1 cup of Kamut, 3 cups of non-dairy milk and bring to boil the way you make oatmeal. Add cinnamon for flavor and cook the oats longer than oatmeal because kamut is firmer in texture.

Cook until you get the texture you desire.

For toppings, add blueberries, strawberries, and baby bananas.

For a sweetener: DO NOT ADD SUGAR.

Use an alkaline gluten-free alternative sweetener called AGAVE to top it off.

What is Agave?

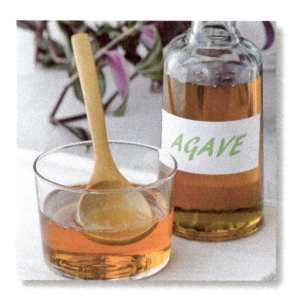

Agave is a gluten free alkaline natural sweetener that comes from the sap of a plant called the century or the maguey, found primarily in Mexico.

What are the benefits of Agave?

It's organic, certified non-GMO, gluten-free, and vegan!

When you use Agave, you are cutting your calories and you achieve the sweetness you desire.

The most important health benefit of Agave is, it has a much lower glycemic index than refined sugar. Agave is also created from natural plant sources.

You can consume Any of these fruits in the morning and throughout the day:

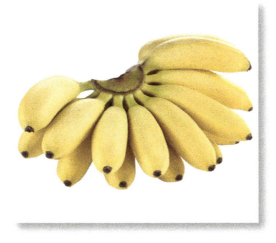

- Apples
- Oranges
- Baby Bananas (Not the really big bananas because they are GMO)
- Blueberries
- Strawberries
- Cantaloupe
- Seeded cherries only
- Seeded grapes only
- Peaches
- Pears
- Plumes
- Prunes
- Seeded raisins only

Note that fruits without any seeds are GMO crops.

Breakfast options 2

2. Parfaits

Non-dairy yogurt, topped with any fruit, granola, nuts, and seeds of choice.

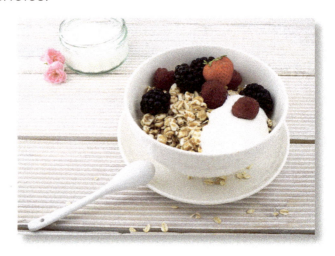

Breakfast options 3

- Turkey bacon
- Turkey sausage
- Salmon - can be used for Croquettes or smoked salmon
- Egg whites
- Chicken Sausage
- Egg white omelets with a lot of vegetables such as peppers, onions, mushrooms, tomatoes, and avocados.

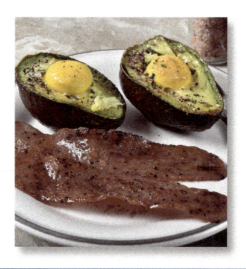

What is GMO?

Here is a straightforward definition of GMO:

"Crops and foods that have been made in a lab versus the crops and foods that God has created for us."

When you are in the process of trying to achieve your desired health and fitness goal, you should also know some breakfast foods to AVOID.

Some of them are listed below:

- Bread unless it is homemade from scratch (gluten-free alkaline bread).
- Waffles
- Pancakes
- Grits
- Oatmeal
- Biscuits
- Toast

All of the above breakfast options pack on weight when you are trying to achieve your health goal.

Lunch:

Eat Lean grilled meats such as:

- Salmon
- Chicken
- Turkey
- Any fish
- Tuna and any Seafood

Eat any of the vegetables below:

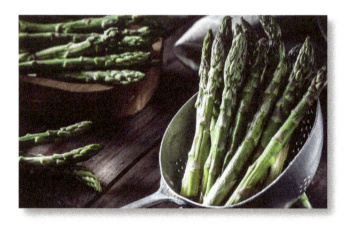

- Asparagus
- Spinach
- Broccoli
- Zucchini
- Squash
- Mushrooms
- Okra
- Olives
- Onions
- Tomatoes (cherry and plum only) non-GMO.
- Turnip greens
- Green/Red/Yellow Peppers
- Lettuce (all except iceberg) which has no nutritional value.

Lunch Foods to AVOID

- Red meats
- Ground beef
- Steaks

Carbohydrates/Starches to Consume:

Carbohydrates are an essential part of your diet. Carbohydrates fuel the body with energy. However, AVOID white carbohydrates such as baked potatoes, mash potatoes, hash browns, French fries, and rice.

Instead of eating white starches, there are alternatives to rice that you can eat while trying to meet your goal.

For instance, quinoa is an alternative to Rice. What is quinoa? It is a gluten-free mineral-rich grain.

KEY: When you cook quinoa, add all-natural ingredients such as garlic powder, onion powder, thyme, pink Himalayan salt, peppers, and onions to taste.

Alternatives to White Starches:

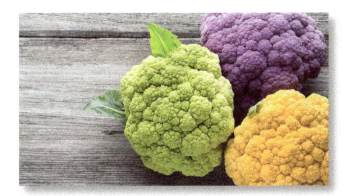

- Cauliflower rice
- Cauliflower mash potatoes
- Complex carbohydrates are used in place of white starches such as Baked sweet potatoes, lentils, and beans.

Dinner:

For dinner, you should always try to eat before 6 pm.

This gives your body time to digest and rest your colon for the night.

For dinner, it is also good to eat a lighter meal before bed.

Salads are very good to eat at night. Keep in mind, Salad dressings contain most of calories, so use sparingly. Limit to two tablespoons of salad dressing.

Vinaigrette salad dressings have less sugar and homemade salad dressings are the best. Here is one of my two homemade salad dressing recipes:

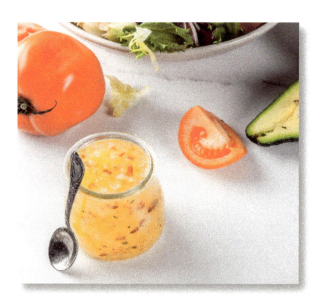

This salad dressing mimics the consistency of ranch dressing:

- ½ cup grape seed oil
- ¼ cup +1 tbsp spring water
- ¼ cup hemp seeds
- 2 tbsp. shallots
- 2 tsp. lime juice
- 1 tsp. onion powder

Use a stick blender to whisk all the ingredients to the consistency you desire. If you want a thicker consistency for dips, do not add a tablespoon of water.

This salad dressing is honey chipotle vinaigrette:

- 1.5 cups grape seed oil
- ½ cup red wine vinegar
- ¼ honey (an alternative is AGAVE which is alkaline and won't raise blood sugar levels for those who are diabetic).
- 3-4 chipotles in adobo
- 4 garlic cloves
- 1 tsp. oregano
- ½ tsp. cumin
- Freshly cracked black pepper
- Squeeze of lime
- Splash of spring water

Salad: Use romaine lettuce instead of iceberg lettuce because it has more nutritional value. Use yellow bell peppers, red bell peppers, and mushrooms. Season your salad with cilantro, thyme, and rosemary. Also add broccoli florets, celery, and carrots to the salad or any raw vegetable to your salad.

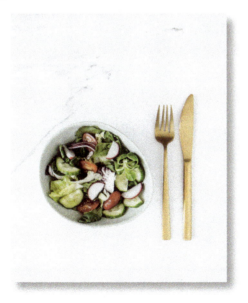

If you have to; you can add eggs and some lean protein to your salad.

Add lean meats on top of your salad such as chicken or any fish. For dinner: Try Lean meats with two servings of vegetables. Avoid taking carbohydrates at night.

Disclaimers: Please consult your medical provider before starting any new meal plan or supplement.

The purpose of this content is to shed some light on some of the key things you can do to jumpstart your health and wellness journey.

I hear people all the time say; I eat right but I don't know why I am not losing any weight. While I was working as a Family Nurse Practitioner in a rural area, I often heard this all the time. I would have one on one sessions with my patients and devote 20-30-minute time slots to focus on breaking their meals down.

I would start by asking, "What do you eat for breakfast?" Some people would say, "I don't eat breakfast." To me, there has been some mixed beliefs on whether or not you should eat breakfast. I usually ask my patients, "Ok, when you don't eat breakfast, when is your first meal?" They would say around 3 o'clock and I would ask, "So what do you eat then?"

They would say; "I eat some chicken, potatoes, green beans and corn." I would then reply by telling them that at least in the morning, even if they don't eat a full breakfast, they should eat a piece of fruit or some crackers to get their metabolism going throughout the day.

Now I know a lot of people engage in intermittent fasting. However, I don't consider this as a lifestyle change but something that people do when they are trying to reach a goal faster. Unfortunately, it often fails at the end when you go back to your original way of eating. My best suggestion is for you to cut out 2 percent of what you do wrong a week – focus on something that makes you feel bad or convicted when you eat it and cut it out of your diet by 2% – and just focus on it this way.

So, for instance, if you drink a Coke or sweet tea with every meal, try cutting out the Coke from one of your meals a week and see how much of a difference it makes with your calorie intake. Another suggestion is, if you eat bread with every meal, such as biscuits or toast for breakfast, cornbread for lunch, and a roll at dinner; A 2% adjustment in your diet would be to cut out the roll at dinner and see how much of a difference it makes with achieving your health and wellness goal.

When I think of a meal plan for my clients, I think of moderation. Moderation is something you don't have to consciously give too much thought to. It's just making the best decision for your overall health choices throughout the day.

On July 4th, I was writing this book and I wanted to include my thought process. So, on July 4th, everyone is usually grilling. So, for instance, everyone loves the typical ribs, macaroni and cheese, baked beans, and banana pudding.

But I had no craving for any of that. I told my husband that we were having grilled salmon, asparagus, zucchini, squash, and spring salad with fruit for dessert. It is a mindset that we have adopted that places food at the forefront of the way we celebrate and fellowship.

On Holidays, fellowship and introduce alternatives and healthier options to your family and friends. Remember Moderation is key!

This example is used to show how being aware of the ingredients in foods is key. Hidden ingredients in foods can stagnate in your health and wellness goals.

So back to the client that skips breakfast and just eats lunch. When I have clients that want to lose weight and have been trying to do everything in their power to eat right, we sit and analyze the ingredients in the food they typically consume. Keep in mind, if you purchased food from a restaurant, there is no way to figure out all the ingredients in it.

But if you cook the food yourself, you know exactly what's in the foods you are eating. Remember this client's meal was Chicken, potatoes, green beans, and corn.

Analysis:

Let's start with the chicken. Chicken typically has steroids and antibiotics in it, unless you select the chicken without it. In fact, the food industry has been destroyed with added preservatives. For instance, steroids make chicken more plumper. Have you ever eaten chicken and you noticed that it's bones were broken, fragile or very dark? This is a sign that the chicken received steroids.

Steroids make the bones in humans and chicken weak. In medicine, we call this osteoporosis – which is brittle bones. Chicken is also given antibiotics because chickens are ill and sick due to some of the substances they are fed. What if I told you, if you can skip eating chicken for one week, you would shed pounds in your face, arms and abdominal area? Something to think about huh?

Now let's just say for instance the corn that was eaten was sprayed with pesticides and other chemicals to make the kernel in the corn large. Spraying the kernel with chemicals is done to make the corn produce more. Corn is considered a GMO which means that it has no nutritional value. Corn is a starch that people see as a vegetable. Corn also raises your blood sugar when eaten.

If you had a vegetable such as green beans, is there protein in it? Does it have white potatoes in it? Was it made with table salt? All of these factors make a huge difference when you are on a journey to discovering why your weight is not reducing despite your efforts.

Is the plate of green beans fresh or canned with a lot of sodium hidden in it?

We know that vegetables are cheap and it is unfortunate the healthier the food is the more expensive it is. A lot of people struggle to pay for food so when shopping select frozen versus canned vegetables to avoid high contents of sodium. Remember, fresh vegetables are always a better choice.

Canned foods typically have about 550-800 mg of sodium content which will ultimately cause inflammation and swelling due to the high sodium content. Sodium also raises blood pressure.

Let's talk about eating foods in a box. Foods in a box contain many preservatives that create a longer shelf life. The longer shelf life makes food last longer and keep the food in place without shifting the contents inside. The preservatives in the food also contain hidden sugars such as high fructose corn syrup.

High Fructose corn syrup sugar content can raise blood sugar 10-20 times higher than regular table sugar. Now let's talk about some of the beverages consumed such as sodas. Sodas have high fructose corn syrup as well as added sugars. In fact, about 50 percent of Sodas are sugar. Beverages such as lemonade, sweet tea, and kool aid are packed with Sugar as well.

Let's say for instance you were able to look at the ingredients in foods and wanted to avoid them, what exactly should you do? You have discovered there are so many preservatives in everything you eat. Here is how you proceed in taking charge of your Nutritional Health.

I suggest that if money is the issue, then try to get frozen vegetables. Try to buy frozen vegetables with one ingredient instead of multiple ingredients. When you look at the pack, for instance, if it is green beans, then make sure the only ingredient is green beans and not green beans and sodium monoxide (a common added preservative).

Did you know being conscious of a 2 % change of the foods you eat is the beginning of subtle changes in your life? These changes are what you can implement daily to help you along the way. I remember when I had a client that suffered from diabetes and could not regulate blood sugars. This client did not want to rely on insulin as well.

After going through the foods that the client was consuming, it was evident that education was needed. The client did not realize most of the sugar being consumed came from drinking sodas. For instance, "All I drink is ginger ale and I love orange and apple juice." Everything is supposed to be done in moderation; nothing is meant to be taken away completely. So let's break down the calories and sugar that are in soda and juices. Ginger ale has 24 grams of sugar. What does that look like?

Sugar/Glucose:

Glucose is the main sugar found in your blood. It is incorporated in foods to provide sweetness.

When you are diabetic, this is one form of sugar that should be avoided unless you have an emergency where you need to bring your blood sugar up due to hypoglycemia (low blood sugar). Under normal circumstances, Glucose in foods should be avoided.

It will spike your blood sugar up and you can easily tell how much sugar you are consuming by looking at your waistline. In medicine, we measure the abdominal area and we call this the abdominal girth. This abdominal girth is a component known as the Metabolic Syndrome. This abdominal girth is a measurement in medicine that is used as a predictor of your cardiovascular and overall health. Metabolic syndrome is a cluster of conditions that increase the risk of heart disease, stroke, and diabetes. It includes high blood pressure, high blood sugar, excess body fat around the waist, and abnormal cholesterol levels. This syndrome increases a person's risk of heart attack and stroke.

Self-care with physical exercise, quitting smoking, weight loss, dietary modification, blood pressure monitoring, cholesterol monitoring, and glucose monitoring are great ways to have an overall analysis of your health.

Another ingredient found in ginger ale is fructose – fructose is a type of sugar that is mostly found in fruits and simple sugars. It contains 50 percent sugar that will spike your blood sugar level if you are diabetic.

Another ingredient in ginger ale is sucrose – sucrose is an artificial sweetener that creates inflammation in the body. How will this inflammation appear in the body? Inflammation presents with swelling, puffiness, and overall weight gain.

Added sugars lead to obesity and spikes in your blood sugar level.

Ginger ale has been a staple in many households when we are sick, nauseated, or to help settle your stomach. This is an exception because when we are sick, we do things to get our bodies back to the point where we feel our best. But Sodas such as Ginger ale should not be a daily drink when trying to reach your health and wellness goals.

Now, what if you love your ginger ale so much that you cannot do without it? What I would suggest is that you make the 2% change.

So, instead of consuming the 16 oz can, adjust to the smaller can of 7.5 oz.

Remember, we never want to cut anything out of our diet cold turkey, instead, we will use the 2 % rule.

Imagine you are cutting back from 16 oz of ginger ale a day to 7.5 oz (which is a smaller can of ginger ale). This implies you will be cutting half of the sugar intake.

Orange juice is another consumable a lot of my clients that suffer from diabetes love. Oranges provide great nutritional value for the body but believe it or not, there are hidden sugars inside of orange juice. The sugar content in orange juice greatly depends on the brand.

Fresh orange juice is the best. Always read the labels. Most of the time, orange juice is concentrated to the point where it has added sugars for a longer shelf life.

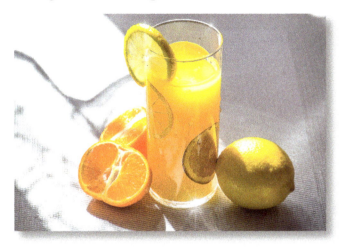

Orange juice is used if your blood sugar is low and you need a boost in sugar during an emergency. But when it comes to your daily consumption, especially if you are struggling with weight gain or diabetes, it is very important you cut 2 % of what you consume each week to help you achieve your desired goal.

A lot of calories we consume come from beverages.

Let's talk about coffee. A health and wellness tip, only add creamer to coffee and do not add any additional sugar. The creamer is already sweetened so there is no need for additional sugar to be added. Table sugar is one of the worst things you can add to your food. I was raised in Memphis, Tennessee and my roots are from Earl, Arkansas.

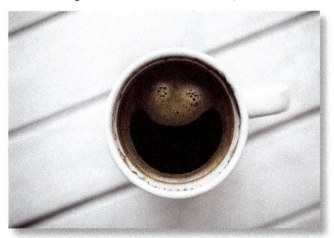

23

We were raised to add sugar on our grits, corn flakes, and cheerios. We drink Kool-Aid with added sugar – almost a half bag of sweetener. When we know better, we do better. So, let's talk about diabetes and sugar and how it affects the body.

Imagine the blood in your body is the source that oxygenates the tissues. Imagine your blood is oxygenated through your veins and arteries and we will use a water hose as an illustration. As blood flows through your body, it is slowed down by the sugars you consume.

Imagine your blood is trying to oxygenate your tissues and it is moving slowly like molasses. It is taking the blood so long to get to your tissues to provide oxygen because there is so much sugar circulating through your body. This leads to a lack of oxygenated tissue in your body.

High sugar content in your blood causes your tissue to be deprived of adequate blood flow. High amounts of sugar in your blood causes the blood and oxygen within to move at a much slower pace. Over time, there is a lot of sugar in the body to the extent that oxygen and blood cannot reach the tissues. This in turn will deprive the body and tissues of essential nutrients. How will it appear on the body? Deprived tissue that lacks oxygen will appear as darkened skin on your legs and limbs such as your shin, feet, and toes, it will also appear as a grey ashy skin tone all over.

If you suffer from diabetes, then you should understand that there are a lot of hidden sugars in boxed foods and sodas. A 2% diet change suggestion would be to avoid eating any food out of a box and limiting sodas. Also, Drink a gallon of water a day.

Water will provide adequate flow of oxygen and blood to all of your organs.

Diabetes

Type 1 Diabetes: This health issue occurs when there is a severe insulin deficiency in the body. The body does not produce insulin from the pancreas. This insulin deficiency causes the body to always be in a high sugar state within. The insulin that comes from the pancreas is destroyed and most clients have to be on insulin with Type 1 Diabetes in order for your body to convert sugars into energy.

Sugar not only comes from sweeteners but also from carbohydrates such as rice, bread, pasta, and potatoes.

Aforementioned, starches are a huge contributor to weight gain and one must use complex carbohydrates instead because they are easily digested and converted from sugars to energy.

Excellent Carbohydrate alternatives include:

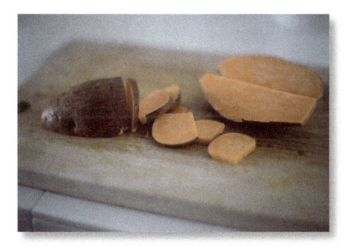

- Quinoa
- Sweet potatoes
- Red potatoes
- Gluten-free flour such as Kamut
- Gluten-free pasta such as Kamut
- Substitution of rice with alternatives such as riced cauliflower.

Type 2 Diabetes: occurs when your body does not use the insulin the body produces to help regulate your blood sugar properly. In type 2 Diabetes the pancreas makes insulin but it is not used properly to break down sugar in the body. What is insulin? Insulin is a hormone produced by the pancreas that helps absorb the sugars in your blood. Whenever your body absorbs sugar, it turns it into energy.

For those with diabetes, their body is not breaking down the sugars; it is storing it as fat instead of energy. This leads to weight gain and affects the entire body by damaging the organs with high sugar levels. When the organs are damaged with high sugar levels, it affects the eyes causing nerve damage, the kidneys causing kidney failure, the tissues causing gangrene, and also leads to overall weight gain.

Glucose levels are Sugar levels that are monitored through your blood.

The current guidelines for monitoring fasting Type II Diabetes sugar levels according to the Art of Science Advanced Practice Nursing recommends that you can randomly check your blood sugar with a portable monitor without eating or drinking for 8 hours or nothing to eat or drink after midnight. The normal level of glucose (sugar) should be between (62-110 mg/dl).

Please consult your Primary Care Provider to know how you can control your blood sugar if you are diagnosed with diabetes.

These parameters are given as a guide for you to know what is the normal range of blood glucose level.

Hypertension

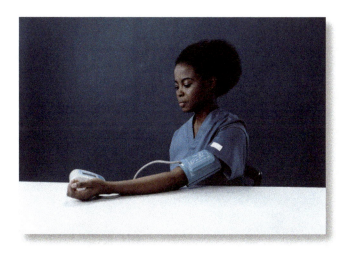

Hypertension "High Blood Pressure" Diet Changes

I am going to explain what high blood pressure is in a more simplified way. Think of the heart like the engine in a car. I like to give analogies and visuals for better understanding. The heart pumps blood throughout your body. Imagine a water hose and I like to use the water hose analogy because it is easier to understand.

A water hose is what the blood flows through. When you have high blood pressure, there is fast-shooting blood that is flowing through the heart and body. The body's blood is supposed to pump with ease and without much "forced" effort. When you have high blood pressure, the pressure inside the water hose will become so fast and high that it forces the blood throughout the body.

This is how you get high blood pressure readings. The blood that is pumping through your body requires a lot of force and when this happens, you feel things such as blurred vision, headaches, shortness of breath, increase in heart rate, and dizziness.

Here are some things you can do to lower your blood pressure naturally. Read your labels and monitor the seasonings in your food.

Particularly seasoning salt and added table salt.

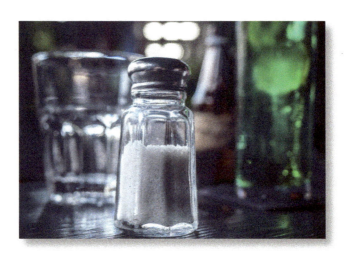

Most of the salts in foods are hidden in ingredients such as monosodium glutamate (MSG). This is an artificial ingredient. What happens with MSG is, salt and water flow together to create an environment for inflammation such as swelling. Swelling is an indicator of inflammation, high salt in the diet, and high blood pressure. This is how salt and water tie into each other.

Salt is made of sodium and chloride. Sodium binds to water in the body and helps maintain the balance of fluids both inside and outside of the cells in the body.

Most meals and foods that have high sodium content are food that are processed or come inside a box such as TV dinners. TV dinners were the worst thing that could have been created because it is quick but most importantly unhealthy and packed with preservatives, artificial meats, and ingredients. TV dinners are also packed with fillers. Fillers are foods that have no nutritional value but are packed with the unknown that swell the stomach creating a full effect only to leave you sluggish.

Source: Eight Joint National Committee (JNC8 Guideline recommends that high blood pressure treatment should start at greater than or equal to 140/90).

Blood pressure goals and recommendations continue to evolve based on new evidence.

According to the 2017 American College of Cardiology/ American heart Associational Guidelines, hypertension is any systolic blood pressure which is the top number greater than or equal to 130 or any diastolic BP measurement bottom number greater than or equal to 80.

Now, what is systolic and diastolic blood pressure?

I want to break this down in simple terms so you can easily understand.

Systolic blood pressure is the amount of blood that pumps through the body when the heart valve opens. Diastolic blood pressure is the amount of blood that fills in the heart before opening. The amount of blood that fills the heart comes at a fast or slow pace. The pace the blood fills the heart cavity is the resting blood pressure which is the bottom number known as diastolic blood pressure.

Here are a few examples of how blood pressure readings are seen:

- (120/80)
- (130/80)
- (140/80)

I tell all my clients to keep a log of their blood pressure either on their phone or a notepad beside the bed to make note of their blood pressure readings . Listen to your body and get to know what you feel like when you have high blood pressure readings or low blood pressure readings. Always jot down the symptoms as well next to the blood pressure.

Start with the date and time of the blood pressure then jot down your blood pressure reading. This is how you can see the trends of how you feel and how your blood pressure is doing. A good diet, exercise, and lots of water throughout the day can help with blood pressure management.

Please consult your Primary Care Provider or Medical Provider for your high blood pressure goals and treatments.

Lifestyle changes in all aspects are essential for your health and some of these changes include but are not limited to:

Here are a few examples of how lifestyle changes can help blood pressure reading:

- Weight loss
- Exercise
- Decreased sodium intake
- DASH diet
- Moderate alcohol consumption
- Smoking Cessation (Quit Smoking)

When you find yourself swelling and have consumed too much salt, you can use dandelion which is a natural diuretic. Diuretics help by eliminating excess fluid and salt in the body by urination.

Dandelion may help reduce water weight, especially when consumed as a dandelion leaf. Dandelion leaves can be sautéed with spinach or any greens with garlic and pepper.

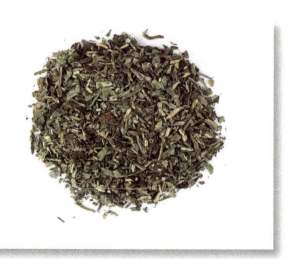

Parsley, is an herb that is known to be a natural diuretic as well as Hibiscus. Can be added to tacos or enchiladas with fresh avocado and pineapple as garnishment. Hibiscus can also be taken as a tea.

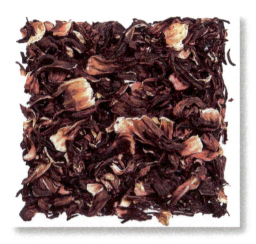

Garlic can be used for flavoring food.

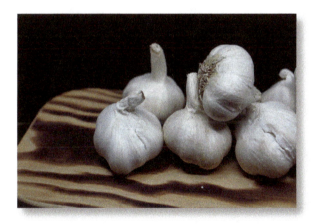

Fennel can be roasted with garlic and grapeseed oil. Fennel is a blub leaf that is crisp in texture and good for salads, pasta, and slaws.

Nettle can be used in a soup with olive oil, vegetables, and dairy-free cream for soups. It can be added to potatoes that are sautéed as well.

Your Health & Water Intake

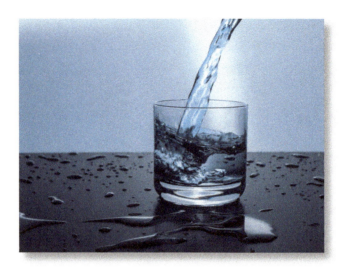

Let's talk about water intake. The human body is about 60 percent water.

The body loses water throughout the day by urinating, sweating, and breathing.

It is recommended that we drink eight bottles of water a day or a gallon a day. Keep in mind factors such as the location we live in and climate also affect the amount of water we need daily.

For instance, if you live in desert areas like Vegas or you live in very hot and humid places, you should consume more water than your average intake.

If your diet consists of coffee and a lot of caffeinated beverages, then your water intake should also increase. Coffees and teas (unless they are decaffeinated) dehydrate you and water should be consumed before and after caffeinated beverages are consumed.

If you are an active person and you exercise a lot, you walk or stand a lot all through your day, then you should drink more water as you engage in more activity.

Dehydration leads to headaches, mood and concentration issues, fatigue, and limited attention focus. Here are some striking benefits of water intake:

- Water intake helps with constipation by liquefying your bowels and helping the foods we eat move throughout our colon.
- Drinking enough water helps you to lose weight because without water, the body can't metabolize fat adequately.
- Water intake helps to flush our kidneys preventing bladder infections and kidney stones.
- Water ensures proper skin hydration. It leaves your skin clearer and helps with acne.
- Water intake maintains the temperature of your body.
- Water lubricates and cushions the joints.

Drink water when you first wake up to help activate your organs and also drink water before a meal to help with digestion.

Carbonated Water

Carbonated water is acidic which may lead to inflammation. Carbonated water also has a lot of sodium content so it is crucial that you read labels and consume in moderation if you love carbonated water.

A lot of people do not really like the taste of water. If you find yourself in this category, then you can increase your water intake through additional means. For instance, you can add some natural fruits and vegetables to your water to give it some flavor and ensure that you consume adequate water intake each day.

Strawberries, blueberries, cucumbers, and lemons are some examples of fruits and vegetables that can add flavor to your water.

You can also add mint leaves and ginger to taste – ginger is very strong so add only a small amount.

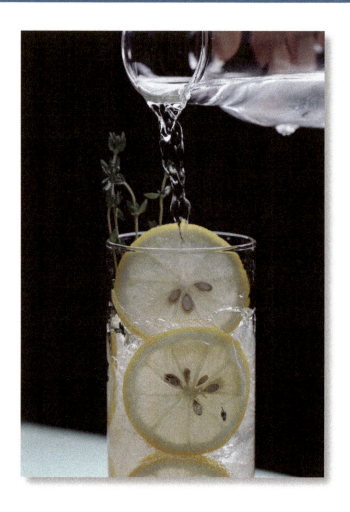

Adding crystal light packages to water I am against. Remember we are reading food labels and all the ingredients we consume. Also, taking a natural approach for sweeteners.

If you use crystal light, use it in moderation and remember, you are not eliminating foods cold turkey; but an introduction to a new lifestyle change that can help you achieve your health and wellness goals. So, focus on changing 2 % of what you are currently doing wrong and begin the implementation of a new lifestyle.

WATER CHART

Body Weight	Daily Requirement	
20 lbs	8 oz.	1 cup
40 lbs	16 oz.	
60 lbs	24 oz.	
80 lbs	32 oz.	4 cups (1/4 gallon or 1 quart)
100 lbs	40 oz.	
120 lbs	48 oz.	
140 lbs	56 oz.	
160 lbs	64 oz.	8 cups (1/2 gallon)
180 lbs	72 oz.	
200 lbs	80 oz.	
220 lbs	88 oz.	
240 lbs	96 oz.	12 cups (3/4 gallon)
260 lbs	104 oz.	
280 lbs	112 oz.	
300 lbs	120 oz.	
320 lbs	128 oz.	16 cups (1 gallon or 4 quarts)

This is a water calculator that will tell you the quantity of water you are supposed to be drinking based on your body weight and height.

According to WebMD, it is recommended that you drink about one ounce of water for each pound that you weigh daily.

For example, I weigh 160 pounds. So, I have to consume 160 ounces of water daily and 160 ounces equals 1.25 gallons of water a day – about 8 -16 oz bottles of water a day.

Here is the converter that will help you understand how much water you are supposed to be drinking a day.

This is how you know you are drinking enough water.

Water Chart:

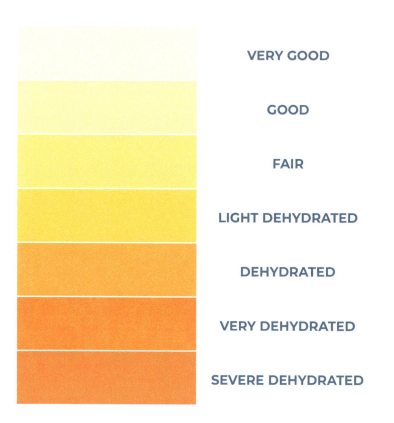

Also, if you go to the restroom every hour to urinate, then you are hydrated. It is the same as a baby that needs his or her diaper changed. You monitor the fluid intake as well as output and that's how you gauge if the baby is hydrated. The same goes for having a number two with bowel habits as babies. But as adults, we forget we were once babies and we have to monitor our output as well.

Cholesterol

According to "Primary Care the Art and Science of Advanced Practice Nursing, 4th edition," the normal range of cholesterol is (120-200/mg).

I am going to break down cholesterol in a simple way in which you will understand. You can think of cholesterol as fat floating around in the body. This fat eventually builds up in the arteries and is deposited in the arteries of your body placing it at risk of heart attacks and strokes. Also, it places you at risk for low blood flow to your legs and feet known as peripheral artery disease.

You might have seen the abbreviation LDL before and it is considered as the "bad" cholesterol in your bloodstream. This bad cholesterol comes from saturated fats in our diet.

High saturated fat content comes from consuming a lot of red meats such as steaks, hamburgers, pork chops, smoked sausages, bacon, and pork sausages.

There are also saturated fats in the snacks we eat such as potato chips, cookies, and donuts.

The normal LDL range is less than 100. Please consult your primary care provider for your goals if you have high cholesterol.

These parameters are given as a general guideline and not tailored individually according to your entire medical history.

Also, you might have seen HDL before and this is the cholesterol that protects your heart from cardiovascular problems such as heart attacks and strokes.

According to Table 10.3, Serum Lipid Levels Caring Based Nursing-The science; normal HDL parameters is optimal to have greater than 60mg/dl reading.

The HDL cholesterol is supposed to be high because it helps to protect the heart. HDL removes excess cholesterol from blood vessels and delivers it back to the liver through reverse cholesterol transport. This will be removed from the liver and released into the intestines as bile. HDL blocks the LDL (which is the bad cholesterol).

Pretty amazing right. So, if you ever go to the doctor to get your lab work done and the doctor tells you that your HDL is low and it is supposed to be high, here are some changes you can make in your diet to help:

- You can consume wild-caught (not farm-raised) fish that has omega 3 to help increase your HDL level.
- Wild-caught salmon, mackerel, tuna, or Omega 3 fish oil over the counter.
- Aerobic activity such as walking and bicycling can help to protect the heart, aid in blood flow and reduce the levels of fat circulating throughout the body.
- Monitor your waistline. For men, it should be less than 40 inches and for women, it should be less than 35 inches.

The waistline is an indicator of how much fat we have in our bodies. In medicine, it is known as "metabolic syndrome."

Metabolic syndrome is a risk calculator that will help you look at your overall health:

1. Abdominal Girth/Abdominal Obesity/Waist Circumference
2. High Triglycerides
3. Reduced HDL
4. High blood pressure
5. Elevated fasting glucose level.

Source: www.americanheart.org/presenter.jhtml?identifier=456

Instead of using margarine, butter, and Crisco that increases cholesterol level, go for alternatives.

Here are some healthier alternative cooking oils:

- Avocado oil
- Brazil nut oil
- Coconut oil (Not made for frying)
- Grapeseed oil
- Hemp seed oil
- Olive oil (Not made for frying)

- Sesame oil
- Walnut oil

Cholesterol content is listed on the ingredients as:

- Saturated Fats
- Trans Fats
- Monosaturated Fats
- Polyunsaturated Fats

Saturated fats are usually seen in meat, butter, and whole milk. The consumption of saturated fats should be between 16-20 grams a day or less.

For consumption based on your health conditions, please consult your primary care provider and dietitian for recommended calorie and nutritional intake.

Trans fat is usually seen in processed foods like TV dinners or boxed foods. They are packed with trans fat for longer shelf life. The key ingredient to avoid is "hydrogenated or partially hydrogenated" oil in these foods.

Monosaturated fats are unsaturated fats and are **recommended** over saturated fats. These types of fats are thought to reduce the bad cholesterol and increase the good cholesterol. Among the best food and recommended food sources of this type of fat include:

- Olive oil
- All plant-based oils
- Nut-based oils
- Sunflower oils
- Cashews
- Popcorn
- Avocados

Lastly, Polyunsaturated fats are typically your Omega 3 foods that are considered to be essential fatty acids. These foods include salmon, sardines, mackerel, other wild-caught fish, beans, legumes, flax, and hemp seeds.

Cholesterol

Here is what high cholesterol means in simplest terms.

Imagine globs of fat floating around in your bloodstream which slows down blood flow to your heart, veins, and arteries. This is what causes heart attacks.

What happens during a heart attack? When a heart attack occurs, fat floats around so much and one day it gets trapped inside the arteries that flow to your heart. In turn, this causes a blocked artery and hinders blood flow to the heart and eventually, a heart attack will occur.

A heart attack is sudden blood flow that cuts off blood circulation in an artery and then the heart muscle starts to die after seconds of impeding blood flow interruption.

This also happens with strokes: except this blood flow problem happened in the blood vessels that travel to the brain. The arteries and veins that allow blood to flow to the brain are shut off by either a blood clot or lack of blood flow particularly plaque – which is fat in the bloodstream from high cholesterol.

There are so many high cholesterol foods we were raised on that are so unhealthy for us.

Here are examples of some of them:

- Crisco cooking oil
- LARD
- Margarine
- Butter

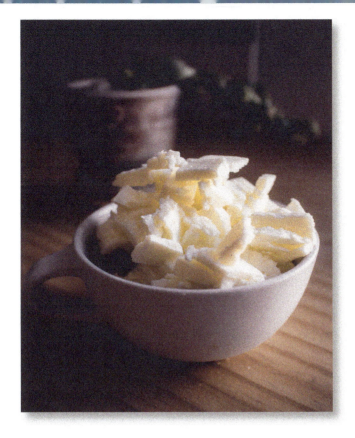

I struggle with cholesterol issues and it is hereditary in my family, so I am very conscious of the fat I eat.

I love fried chicken, fried catfish, french fries, and more. But the truth of the matter is, it has to be in moderation. I cannot consume fried foods every day, but only once in a while. Remember a 2% dietary change.

It's not only fried foods that have hidden fat; it is in snacks particularly crackers, chips, as well as condiments.

Hidden Ingredient Soybean Oil raises cholesterol levels. This is a NO-NO. You can find this in peanut butter or cheese crackers, condiments such as Mayo, and a lot of salad dressings. Soybean oil raises your cholesterol levels 10-20 times higher in the blood.

Conclusion

I want to personally congratulate you for investing in your health and wellness! I hope this book was enlightening and provided useful information on 2 % of things that could be changed to take your health to the next level. I hope that I was able to provide great value in the content of this book.

You will find attached a 30-day meal tracker along with a weight, inch, and water intake tracker.

Remember this is not a quick fad; this is implementing a 2% change in what you incorporate into your new lifestyle. The goal of making just a 2 % change is to ensure that you can adapt to a new lifestyle without feeling stressed or overwhelmed.

All it takes is making just a 2% change. It does not matter when you start; what matters is that you start the process. This 30-day tracker will be a guide for you to see your progress and what you implemented in your 30-day 2 % change. Here are a few health tips to further assist you in your journey.

Health Tip 1:

The stomach is the size of a large fist but it can stretched and expanded. When we stretch the stomach, we force more food into it to the point where we are FULL. Don't eat to get full; eat to give the body the essential nutrients it needs. For example, when you fix your plate, add a lot of fruits and vegetables and eat those first so you can ensure your body has the fuel and nutrients it needs. Then migrate to protein and carbohydrates.

Health Tip 2:

When you fix your plate, use a smaller plate like a saucer. Using a smaller plate will allow you to see the amount of food that fits into your stomach without overstuffing or getting really FULL. When you feel your stomach is getting full, simply stop eating, drink some water and you're DONE.

Food Journal

Month : _____

Write your meals & cups of water intake.

MEALS	MONDAY	TUESDAY	WEDNESDAY
WEEK 1 BREAKFAST			
LUNCH			
DINNER			

MEALS	MONDAY	TUESDAY	WEDNESDAY
WEEK 2 BREAKFAST			
LUNCH			
DINNER			

MEALS	MONDAY	TUESDAY	WEDNESDAY
WEEK 3 BREAKFAST			
LUNCH			
DINNER			

MEALS	MONDAY	TUESDAY	WEDNESDAY
WEEK 4 BREAKFAST			
LUNCH			
DINNER			

Food Journal

Write your meals & cups of water intake.

THURSDAY	FRIDAY	SATURDAY	SUNDAY

Exercise Journal

Month : _____

WEEK 1	WEEK 2	WEEK 3	WEEK 4

Workout:

Duration:

Calories Burned :

Workout:

Duration:

Calories Burned :

Workout:

Duration:

Calories Burned :

Workout:

Duration:

Calories Burned :

Workout:

Duration:

Calories Burned :

Workout:

Duration:

Calories Burned :

Workout:

Duration:

Calories Burned :

Progress Report

Month : _____

How was I successful?

How do I feel?

What didn't go so well?

What motivates me?

What can I do Differently?

Previous Weight: _____

Current Weight: _____

Inches:

Previous Waist Circumference: _____

Current Waist Circumference: _____

I give myself :

☆ ☆ ☆ ☆ ☆

Food Journal

Month : _____

Write your meals & cups of water intake.

	MEALS	MONDAY	TUESDAY	WEDNESDAY
WEEK 1	BREAKFAST			
	LUNCH			
	DINNER			
WEEK 2	BREAKFAST			
	LUNCH			
	DINNER			
WEEK 3	BREAKFAST			
	LUNCH			
	DINNER			
WEEK 4	BREAKFAST			
	LUNCH			
	DINNER			

Food Journal

Write your meals & cups of water intake.

THURSDAY	FRIDAY	SATURDAY	SUNDAY

Exercise Journal

Month : _____

WEEK 1	WEEK 2	WEEK 3	WEEK 4
Workout: Duration: Calories Burned :	Workout: Duration: Calories Burned :	Workout: Duration: Calories Burned :	Workout: Duration: Calories Burned :
Workout: Duration: Calories Burned :	Workout: Duration: Calories Burned :	Workout: Duration: Calories Burned :	Workout: Duration: Calories Burned :
Workout: Duration: Calories Burned :	Workout: Duration: Calories Burned :	Workout: Duration: Calories Burned :	Workout: Duration: Calories Burned :
Workout: Duration: Calories Burned :	Workout: Duration: Calories Burned :	Workout: Duration: Calories Burned :	Workout: Duration: Calories Burned :
Workout: Duration: Calories Burned :	Workout: Duration: Calories Burned :	Workout: Duration: Calories Burned :	Workout: Duration: Calories Burned :
Workout: Duration: Calories Burned :	Workout: Duration: Calories Burned :	Workout: Duration: Calories Burned :	Workout: Duration: Calories Burned :
Workout: Duration: Calories Burned :	Workout: Duration: Calories Burned :	Workout: Duration: Calories Burned :	Workout: Duration: Calories Burned :

Progress Report

Month : _____

How was I successful?

How do I feel?

What didn't go so well?

What motivates me?

What can I do Differently?

Previous Weight:_____

Current Weight: _____

Inches:

Previous Waist Circumference: _____

Current Waist Circumference: _____

I give myself :

☆ ☆ ☆ ☆ ☆

Food Journal

Month : _____

Write your meals & cups of water intake.

MEALS	MONDAY	TUESDAY	WEDNESDAY
WEEK 1 BREAKFAST			
LUNCH			
DINNER			

MEALS	MONDAY	TUESDAY	WEDNESDAY
WEEK 2 BREAKFAST			
LUNCH			
DINNER			

MEALS	MONDAY	TUESDAY	WEDNESDAY
WEEK 3 BREAKFAST			
LUNCH			
DINNER			

MEALS	MONDAY	TUESDAY	WEDNESDAY
WEEK 4 BREAKFAST			
LUNCH			
DINNER			

Food Journal

Write your meals & cups of water intake.

THURSDAY	FRIDAY	SATURDAY	SUNDAY

Exercise Journal

Month : _____

WEEK 1	WEEK 2	WEEK 3	WEEK 4
Workout: Duration: Calories Burned :	Workout: Duration: Calories Burned :	Workout: Duration: Calories Burned :	Workout: Duration: Calories Burned :
Workout: Duration: Calories Burned :	Workout: Duration: Calories Burned :	Workout: Duration: Calories Burned :	Workout: Duration: Calories Burned :
Workout: Duration: Calories Burned :	Workout: Duration: Calories Burned :	Workout: Duration: Calories Burned :	Workout: Duration: Calories Burned :
Workout: Duration: Calories Burned :	Workout: Duration: Calories Burned :	Workout: Duration: Calories Burned :	Workout: Duration: Calories Burned :
Workout: Duration: Calories Burned :	Workout: Duration: Calories Burned :	Workout: Duration: Calories Burned :	Workout: Duration: Calories Burned :
Workout: Duration: Calories Burned :	Workout: Duration: Calories Burned :	Workout: Duration: Calories Burned :	Workout: Duration: Calories Burned :
Workout: Duration: Calories Burned :	Workout: Duration: Calories Burned :	Workout: Duration: Calories Burned :	Workout: Duration: Calories Burned :

Progress Report

Month : _____

How was I successful?

How do I feel?

What didn't go so well?

What motivates me?

What can I do Differently?

Previous Weight: _____

Current Weight: _____

Inches:

Previous Waist Circumference: _____

Current Waist Circumference: _____

I give myself :

☆ ☆ ☆ ☆ ☆

Food Journal

Month : _____

Write your meals & cups of water intake.

MEALS		MONDAY	TUESDAY	WEDNESDAY
WEEK 1	BREAKFAST			
	LUNCH			
	DINNER			
WEEK 2	BREAKFAST			
	LUNCH			
	DINNER			
WEEK 3	BREAKFAST			
	LUNCH			
	DINNER			
WEEK 4	BREAKFAST			
	LUNCH			
	DINNER			

Food Journal

Write your meals & cups of water intake.

THURSDAY	FRIDAY	SATURDAY	SUNDAY

Exercise Journal

Month : _____

WEEK 1	WEEK 2	WEEK 3	WEEK 4
Workout: Duration: Calories Burned :	Workout: Duration: Calories Burned :	Workout: Duration: Calories Burned :	Workout: Duration: Calories Burned :
Workout: Duration: Calories Burned :	Workout: Duration: Calories Burned :	Workout: Duration: Calories Burned :	Workout: Duration: Calories Burned :
Workout: Duration: Calories Burned :	Workout: Duration: Calories Burned :	Workout: Duration: Calories Burned :	Workout: Duration: Calories Burned :
Workout: Duration: Calories Burned :	Workout: Duration: Calories Burned :	Workout: Duration: Calories Burned :	Workout: Duration: Calories Burned :
Workout: Duration: Calories Burned :	Workout: Duration: Calories Burned :	Workout: Duration: Calories Burned :	Workout: Duration: Calories Burned :
Workout: Duration: Calories Burned :	Workout: Duration: Calories Burned :	Workout: Duration: Calories Burned :	Workout: Duration: Calories Burned :
Workout: Duration: Calories Burned :	Workout: Duration: Calories Burned :	Workout: Duration: Calories Burned :	Workout: Duration: Calories Burned :

Progress Report

Month : _____

How was I successful?

How do I feel?

What didn't go so well?

What motivates me?

What can I do Differently?

Previous Weight: _____

Current Weight: _____

Inches:

Previous Waist Circumference: _____

Current Waist Circumference: _____

I give myself :

☆ ☆ ☆ ☆ ☆

Food Journal

Month : _____

Write your meals & cups of water intake.

	MEALS	MONDAY	TUESDAY	WEDNESDAY
WEEK 1	BREAKFAST			
	LUNCH			
	DINNER			
WEEK 2	BREAKFAST			
	LUNCH			
	DINNER			
WEEK 3	BREAKFAST			
	LUNCH			
	DINNER			
WEEK 4	BREAKFAST			
	LUNCH			
	DINNER			

Food Journal

Write your meals & cups of water intake.

THURSDAY	FRIDAY	SATURDAY	SUNDAY

Exercise Journal

Month : _____

WEEK 1	WEEK 2	WEEK 3	WEEK 4
Workout: Duration: Calories Burned :	Workout: Duration: Calories Burned :	Workout: Duration: Calories Burned :	Workout: Duration: Calories Burned :
Workout: Duration: Calories Burned :	Workout: Duration: Calories Burned :	Workout: Duration: Calories Burned :	Workout: Duration: Calories Burned :
Workout: Duration: Calories Burned :	Workout: Duration: Calories Burned :	Workout: Duration: Calories Burned :	Workout: Duration: Calories Burned :
Workout: Duration: Calories Burned :	Workout: Duration: Calories Burned :	Workout: Duration: Calories Burned :	Workout: Duration: Calories Burned :
Workout: Duration: Calories Burned :	Workout: Duration: Calories Burned :	Workout: Duration: Calories Burned :	Workout: Duration: Calories Burned :
Workout: Duration: Calories Burned :	Workout: Duration: Calories Burned :	Workout: Duration: Calories Burned :	Workout: Duration: Calories Burned :
Workout: Duration: Calories Burned :	Workout: Duration: Calories Burned :	Workout: Duration: Calories Burned :	Workout: Duration: Calories Burned :

Progress Report

Month : _____

How was I successful?

How do I feel?

What didn't go so well?

What motivates me?

What can I do Differently?

Previous Weight: _____

Current Weight: _____

Inches:

Previous Waist Circumference: _____

Current Waist Circumference: _____

I give myself :

☆ ☆ ☆ ☆ ☆

Food Journal

Month : _____

Write your meals & cups of water intake.

	MEALS	MONDAY	TUESDAY	WEDNESDAY
WEEK 1	BREAKFAST			
	LUNCH			
	DINNER			
	🥛🥛🥛🥛🥛🥛🥛🥛			
WEEK 2	BREAKFAST			
	LUNCH			
	DINNER			
	🥛🥛🥛🥛🥛🥛🥛🥛			
WEEK 3	BREAKFAST			
	LUNCH			
	DINNER			
	🥛🥛🥛🥛🥛🥛🥛🥛			
WEEK 4	BREAKFAST			
	LUNCH			
	DINNER			
	🥛🥛🥛🥛🥛🥛🥛🥛			

Food Journal

Write your meals & cups of water intake.

THURSDAY	FRIDAY	SATURDAY	SUNDAY

Exercise Journal

Month : _____

WEEK 1	WEEK 2	WEEK 3	WEEK 4
Workout: Duration: Calories Burned :	Workout: Duration: Calories Burned :	Workout: Duration: Calories Burned :	Workout: Duration: Calories Burned :
Workout: Duration: Calories Burned :	Workout: Duration: Calories Burned :	Workout: Duration: Calories Burned :	Workout: Duration: Calories Burned :
Workout: Duration: Calories Burned :	Workout: Duration: Calories Burned :	Workout: Duration: Calories Burned :	Workout: Duration: Calories Burned :
Workout: Duration: Calories Burned :	Workout: Duration: Calories Burned :	Workout: Duration: Calories Burned :	Workout: Duration: Calories Burned :
Workout: Duration: Calories Burned :	Workout: Duration: Calories Burned :	Workout: Duration: Calories Burned :	Workout: Duration: Calories Burned :
Workout: Duration: Calories Burned :	Workout: Duration: Calories Burned :	Workout: Duration: Calories Burned :	Workout: Duration: Calories Burned :
Workout: Duration: Calories Burned :	Workout: Duration: Calories Burned :	Workout: Duration: Calories Burned :	Workout: Duration: Calories Burned :

Progress Report

Month : _____

How was I successful?

How do I feel?

What didn't go so well?

What motivates me?

What can I do Differently?

Previous Weight: _____

Current Weight: _____

Inches:

Previous Waist Circumference: _____

Current Waist Circumference: _____

I give myself :

☆ ☆ ☆ ☆ ☆

Food Journal

Month : _____

Write your meals & cups of water intake.

	MEALS	MONDAY	TUESDAY	WEDNESDAY
WEEK 1	BREAKFAST			
	LUNCH			
	DINNER			
WEEK 2	BREAKFAST			
	LUNCH			
	DINNER			
WEEK 3	BREAKFAST			
	LUNCH			
	DINNER			
WEEK 4	BREAKFAST			
	LUNCH			
	DINNER			

Food Journal

Write your meals & cups of water intake.

THURSDAY	FRIDAY	SATURDAY	SUNDAY

Exercise Journal

Month : _____

WEEK 1	WEEK 2	WEEK 3	WEEK 4
Workout: Duration: Calories Burned :	Workout: Duration: Calories Burned :	Workout: Duration: Calories Burned :	Workout: Duration: Calories Burned :
Workout: Duration: Calories Burned :	Workout: Duration: Calories Burned :	Workout: Duration: Calories Burned :	Workout: Duration: Calories Burned :
Workout: Duration: Calories Burned :	Workout: Duration: Calories Burned :	Workout: Duration: Calories Burned :	Workout: Duration: Calories Burned :
Workout: Duration: Calories Burned :	Workout: Duration: Calories Burned :	Workout: Duration: Calories Burned :	Workout: Duration: Calories Burned :
Workout: Duration: Calories Burned :	Workout: Duration: Calories Burned :	Workout: Duration: Calories Burned :	Workout: Duration: Calories Burned :
Workout: Duration: Calories Burned :	Workout: Duration: Calories Burned :	Workout: Duration: Calories Burned :	Workout: Duration: Calories Burned :
Workout: Duration: Calories Burned :	Workout: Duration: Calories Burned :	Workout: Duration: Calories Burned :	Workout: Duration: Calories Burned :

Progress Report

Month : _____

How was I successful?

How do I feel?

What didn't go so well?

What motivates me?

What can I do Differently?

Previous Weight: _____

Current Weight: _____

Inches:

Previous Waist Circumference: _____

Current Waist Circumference: _____

I give myself :

☆ ☆ ☆ ☆ ☆

Food Journal

Month : _____

Write your meals & cups of water intake.

MEALS	MONDAY	TUESDAY	WEDNESDAY
WEEK 1 BREAKFAST			
LUNCH			
DINNER			

MEALS	MONDAY	TUESDAY	WEDNESDAY
WEEK 2 BREAKFAST			
LUNCH			
DINNER			

MEALS	MONDAY	TUESDAY	WEDNESDAY
WEEK 3 BREAKFAST			
LUNCH			
DINNER			

MEALS	MONDAY	TUESDAY	WEDNESDAY
WEEK 4 BREAKFAST			
LUNCH			
DINNER			

Food Journal

Write your meals & cups of water intake.

THURSDAY	FRIDAY	SATURDAY	SUNDAY

Exercise Journal

Month : _____

WEEK 1	WEEK 2	WEEK 3	WEEK 4
Workout: Duration: Calories Burned :	Workout: Duration: Calories Burned :	Workout: Duration: Calories Burned :	Workout: Duration: Calories Burned :
Workout: Duration: Calories Burned :	Workout: Duration: Calories Burned :	Workout: Duration: Calories Burned :	Workout: Duration: Calories Burned :
Workout: Duration: Calories Burned :	Workout: Duration: Calories Burned :	Workout: Duration: Calories Burned :	Workout: Duration: Calories Burned :
Workout: Duration: Calories Burned :	Workout: Duration: Calories Burned :	Workout: Duration: Calories Burned :	Workout: Duration: Calories Burned :
Workout: Duration: Calories Burned :	Workout: Duration: Calories Burned :	Workout: Duration: Calories Burned :	Workout: Duration: Calories Burned :
Workout: Duration: Calories Burned :	Workout: Duration: Calories Burned :	Workout: Duration: Calories Burned :	Workout: Duration: Calories Burned :
Workout: Duration: Calories Burned :	Workout: Duration: Calories Burned :	Workout: Duration: Calories Burned :	Workout: Duration: Calories Burned :

Progress Report

Month : _____

How was I successful?

How do I feel?

What didn't go so well?

What motivates me?

What can I do Differently?

Previous Weight: _____

Current Weight: _____

Inches:

Previous Waist Circumference: _____

Current Waist Circumference: _____

I give myself :

☆ ☆ ☆ ☆ ☆

Food Journal

Month : _____

Write your meals & cups of water intake.

MEALS		MONDAY	TUESDAY	WEDNESDAY
WEEK 1	BREAKFAST			
	LUNCH			
	DINNER			

MEALS		MONDAY	TUESDAY	WEDNESDAY
WEEK 2	BREAKFAST			
	LUNCH			
	DINNER			

MEALS		MONDAY	TUESDAY	WEDNESDAY
WEEK 3	BREAKFAST			
	LUNCH			
	DINNER			

MEALS		MONDAY	TUESDAY	WEDNESDAY
WEEK 4	BREAKFAST			
	LUNCH			
	DINNER			

Food Journal

Write your meals & cups of water intake.

THURSDAY	FRIDAY	SATURDAY	SUNDAY

Exercise Journal

Month : _____

WEEK 1	WEEK 2	WEEK 3	WEEK 4
Workout: Duration: Calories Burned :	Workout: Duration: Calories Burned :	Workout: Duration: Calories Burned :	Workout: Duration: Calories Burned :
Workout: Duration: Calories Burned :	Workout: Duration: Calories Burned :	Workout: Duration: Calories Burned :	Workout: Duration: Calories Burned :
Workout: Duration: Calories Burned :	Workout: Duration: Calories Burned :	Workout: Duration: Calories Burned :	Workout: Duration: Calories Burned :
Workout: Duration: Calories Burned :	Workout: Duration: Calories Burned :	Workout: Duration: Calories Burned :	Workout: Duration: Calories Burned :
Workout: Duration: Calories Burned :	Workout: Duration: Calories Burned :	Workout: Duration: Calories Burned :	Workout: Duration: Calories Burned :
Workout: Duration: Calories Burned :	Workout: Duration: Calories Burned :	Workout: Duration: Calories Burned :	Workout: Duration: Calories Burned :
Workout: Duration: Calories Burned :	Workout: Duration: Calories Burned :	Workout: Duration: Calories Burned :	Workout: Duration: Calories Burned :

Progress Report

Month : _____

How was I successful?

How do I feel?

What didn't go so well?

What motivates me?

What can I do Differently?

Previous Weight: _____

Current Weight: _____

Inches:

Previous Waist Circumference: _____

Current Waist Circumference: _____

I give myself :

☆ ☆ ☆ ☆ ☆

Food Journal

Month : _____

Write your meals & cups of water intake.

	MEALS	MONDAY	TUESDAY	WEDNESDAY
WEEK 1	BREAKFAST			
	LUNCH			
	DINNER			

WEEK 2	BREAKFAST			
	LUNCH			
	DINNER			

WEEK 3	BREAKFAST			
	LUNCH			
	DINNER			

WEEK 4	BREAKFAST			
	LUNCH			
	DINNER			

Food Journal

Write your meals & cups of water intake.

THURSDAY	FRIDAY	SATURDAY	SUNDAY

Exercise Journal

Month : _____

WEEK 1	WEEK 2	WEEK 3	WEEK 4
Workout: Duration: Calories Burned :	Workout: Duration: Calories Burned :	Workout: Duration: Calories Burned :	Workout: Duration: Calories Burned :
Workout: Duration: Calories Burned :	Workout: Duration: Calories Burned :	Workout: Duration: Calories Burned :	Workout: Duration: Calories Burned :
Workout: Duration: Calories Burned :	Workout: Duration: Calories Burned :	Workout: Duration: Calories Burned :	Workout: Duration: Calories Burned :
Workout: Duration: Calories Burned :	Workout: Duration: Calories Burned :	Workout: Duration: Calories Burned :	Workout: Duration: Calories Burned :
Workout: Duration: Calories Burned :	Workout: Duration: Calories Burned :	Workout: Duration: Calories Burned :	Workout: Duration: Calories Burned :
Workout: Duration: Calories Burned :	Workout: Duration: Calories Burned :	Workout: Duration: Calories Burned :	Workout: Duration: Calories Burned :
Workout: Duration: Calories Burned :	Workout: Duration: Calories Burned :	Workout: Duration: Calories Burned :	Workout: Duration: Calories Burned :

Progress Report

Month : _____

How was I successful?

How do I feel?

What didn't go so well?

What motivates me?

What can I do Differently?

Previous Weight: _____

Current Weight: _____

Inches:

Previous Waist Circumference: _____

Current Waist Circumference: _____

I give myself :

☆ ☆ ☆ ☆ ☆

Food Journal

Month : _____

Write your meals & cups of water intake.

	MEALS	MONDAY	TUESDAY	WEDNESDAY
WEEK 1	BREAKFAST			
	LUNCH			
	DINNER			
WEEK 2	BREAKFAST			
	LUNCH			
	DINNER			
WEEK 3	BREAKFAST			
	LUNCH			
	DINNER			
WEEK 4	BREAKFAST			
	LUNCH			
	DINNER			

Food Journal

Write your meals & cups of water intake.

THURSDAY	FRIDAY	SATURDAY	SUNDAY

Exercise Journal

Month : _____

WEEK 1	WEEK 2	WEEK 3	WEEK 4
Workout: Duration: Calories Burned :	Workout: Duration: Calories Burned :	Workout: Duration: Calories Burned :	Workout: Duration: Calories Burned :
Workout: Duration: Calories Burned :	Workout: Duration: Calories Burned :	Workout: Duration: Calories Burned :	Workout: Duration: Calories Burned :
Workout: Duration: Calories Burned :	Workout: Duration: Calories Burned :	Workout: Duration: Calories Burned :	Workout: Duration: Calories Burned :
Workout: Duration: Calories Burned :	Workout: Duration: Calories Burned :	Workout: Duration: Calories Burned :	Workout: Duration: Calories Burned :
Workout: Duration: Calories Burned :	Workout: Duration: Calories Burned :	Workout: Duration: Calories Burned :	Workout: Duration: Calories Burned :
Workout: Duration: Calories Burned :	Workout: Duration: Calories Burned :	Workout: Duration: Calories Burned :	Workout: Duration: Calories Burned :
Workout: Duration: Calories Burned :	Workout: Duration: Calories Burned :	Workout: Duration: Calories Burned :	Workout: Duration: Calories Burned :

Progress Report

Month : _____

How was I successful?

How do I feel?

What didn't go so well?

What motivates me?

What can I do Differently?

Previous Weight: _____

Current Weight: _____

Inches:

Previous Waist Circumference: _____

Current Waist Circumference: _____

I give myself :

☆ ☆ ☆ ☆ ☆

Food Journal

Month : _____

Write your meals & cups of water intake.

	MEALS	MONDAY	TUESDAY	WEDNESDAY
WEEK 1	BREAKFAST			
	LUNCH			
	DINNER			
WEEK 2	BREAKFAST			
	LUNCH			
	DINNER			
WEEK 3	BREAKFAST			
	LUNCH			
	DINNER			
WEEK 4	BREAKFAST			
	LUNCH			
	DINNER			

Food Journal

Write your meals & cups of water intake.

THURSDAY	FRIDAY	SATURDAY	SUNDAY

Exercise Journal

Month : _____

WEEK 1	WEEK 2	WEEK 3	WEEK 4
Workout: Duration: Calories Burned :	Workout: Duration: Calories Burned :	Workout: Duration: Calories Burned :	Workout: Duration: Calories Burned :
Workout: Duration: Calories Burned :	Workout: Duration: Calories Burned :	Workout: Duration: Calories Burned :	Workout: Duration: Calories Burned :
Workout: Duration: Calories Burned :	Workout: Duration: Calories Burned :	Workout: Duration: Calories Burned :	Workout: Duration: Calories Burned :
Workout: Duration: Calories Burned :	Workout: Duration: Calories Burned :	Workout: Duration: Calories Burned :	Workout: Duration: Calories Burned :
Workout: Duration: Calories Burned :	Workout: Duration: Calories Burned :	Workout: Duration: Calories Burned :	Workout: Duration: Calories Burned :
Workout: Duration: Calories Burned :	Workout: Duration: Calories Burned :	Workout: Duration: Calories Burned :	Workout: Duration: Calories Burned :
Workout: Duration: Calories Burned :	Workout: Duration: Calories Burned :	Workout: Duration: Calories Burned :	Workout: Duration: Calories Burned :

Progress Report

Month : _____

How was I successful?

How do I feel?

What didn't go so well?

What motivates me?

What can I do Differently?

Previous Weight: _____

Current Weight: _____

Inches:

Previous Waist Circumference: _____

Current Waist Circumference: _____

I give myself :

☆ ☆ ☆ ☆ ☆

List of Preservatives in Foods:

Acesulfame K
(Acesulfame Potassium)
Alum) Aluminum Ammonium Sulfate
Ammonium Chloride
Artificial Colors
Artificial Flavors
Aspartame
Astaxanthin
Autolyzed yeast Extract
Azo Dyes
Azodicarbonamide
Benzoic Acid
Benzyl Alcohol/Benzoyl Peroxide
BHA (Butylated Hydroxytoluene
BHT Butylated Hydroxytoluene
Bromated Flour
Brominated Vegetable Oil
Calcium Bromate
Calcium Peroxide
Calcium Sorbate
Canthaxanthin
Caprocaprylobehe9n
Carmel Flavor
Carboxymethyl Cellulose
Carmine/Cochineal
DATEM (Diacetyl Tartaric Acid)
Diacetyl/Acetoin
Dipotassium Sulfate
Disodium Inosinate
EDTA Calcium Disodium EDTA
Esters of Fatty Acids
Ethoxyquin
Fat Substitutes (Sucrose Polyester)
Glycerides
Glycerol
High Fructose corn syrup
Hydrogenated Starch
Hydrolyzed Soy or Corn Protein
Lard or Crisco
L-Cysteine
Maltodextrin

Monosodium Glutamate/Sodium Glutamate – *causes high blood pressure and inflammation*
Neotame
Nitrates seen in hot dogs, cause headaches
Paraben
Partially Hydrogenated oils
Polydextrose
Polyethylene glycol (PEG)
Polysorbates
Potassium Benzoate
Potassium Bisulfate
Potassium Lactate
Potassium Sorbate
Propionates
Propionic Acid
Propylene Glycol
Propylene Glycol Alginate
Saccharin
Salatrim
Silicates/Bentonite
Silicone/Siloxanes
Artificial Smoke Flavor
Sodium Benzoate
Sodium Diacetate
Sodium Erythorbate
Sodium Lactate
Sodium Lauryl Sulfate
Sodium Metabisulfite
Sodium Phosphate
Disodium Phosphate
Trisodium Phosphate
Sorbates
Sorbic Acid
Stannous Chloride
Sucralose
Sucroglycerides
Sulfites
Sulfur Dioxide
Tertiary TBHQ Butylhydroquinone
Theobromine
Titanium Dioxide
Triacetin/Glycerol
Vanillin

References:

Sources: Dunphy, M. Lynn, Brown, Windland E. Jill, Porter O. Brian, Thomas J Debera Primary Care the Art and Science of Advanced Practice Nursing, 4th edition.

Sources/References: The Eighth Joint National Committee (JNC8) guidelines, 2017 American College of Cardiology/American Heart Association. Epocrates Guidelines, Dunphy, Lynne M, Brown Winland E. Jill, Porter Brian O, Thomas J. Debra primary care the art of science of advanced practice nursing 4th edition.

About the Author

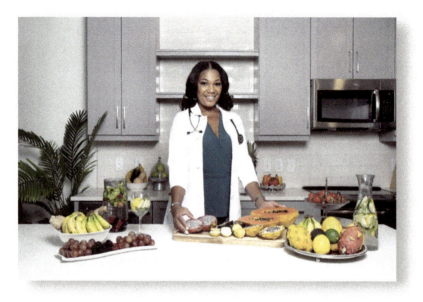

Crystal Branch was born in Memphis, Tennessee. She obtained a Bachelor's of Science in Nursing from the University of Memphis and became a Nurse Practitioner with a Master's Degree in Science from Barry University. Crystal's Tenure includes: Multispecialty Experience in Neonates, Maternity, Pediatric, Adults, and Geriatric Patient Population, Multispecialty Experience in Cardiology, Medical-Surgical, Orthopedics, Neurology, Psychiatric, Rehabilitation and Pain Management, Urgent Care, and Primary Care.

Crystal's passion is to educate and enlighten her community on Nutritional Health as it relates to Chronic Conditions and Weight Management and as a result she started her own Coaching Program Business where she helps individuals reach their health, wellness and weight loss goals. Crystal also provides business coaching, life coaching, and mentorship.

Crystal resides in Atlanta, GA, is married and working on starting a family. Crystal enjoys traveling, dancing, singing, cooking, and spending time with her family and friends.

For more information visit: www.purposeinpain.global

Email: PurposeinPain2021@gmail.com

SCAN TO VISIT MY WEBSITE

Interested in Writing and/or Publishing Book?
Contact Dr. Synovia @ a2zbookspublishing.net
or @Dr.Synovia on Instagram.

CPSIA information can be obtained
at www.ICGtesting.com
Printed in the USA
LVHW070305060422
715340LV00010B/422